How Many People Does It Take To Make A Baby?

Amazing donors and surrogates can help build a family

By Kelly and John Sparry

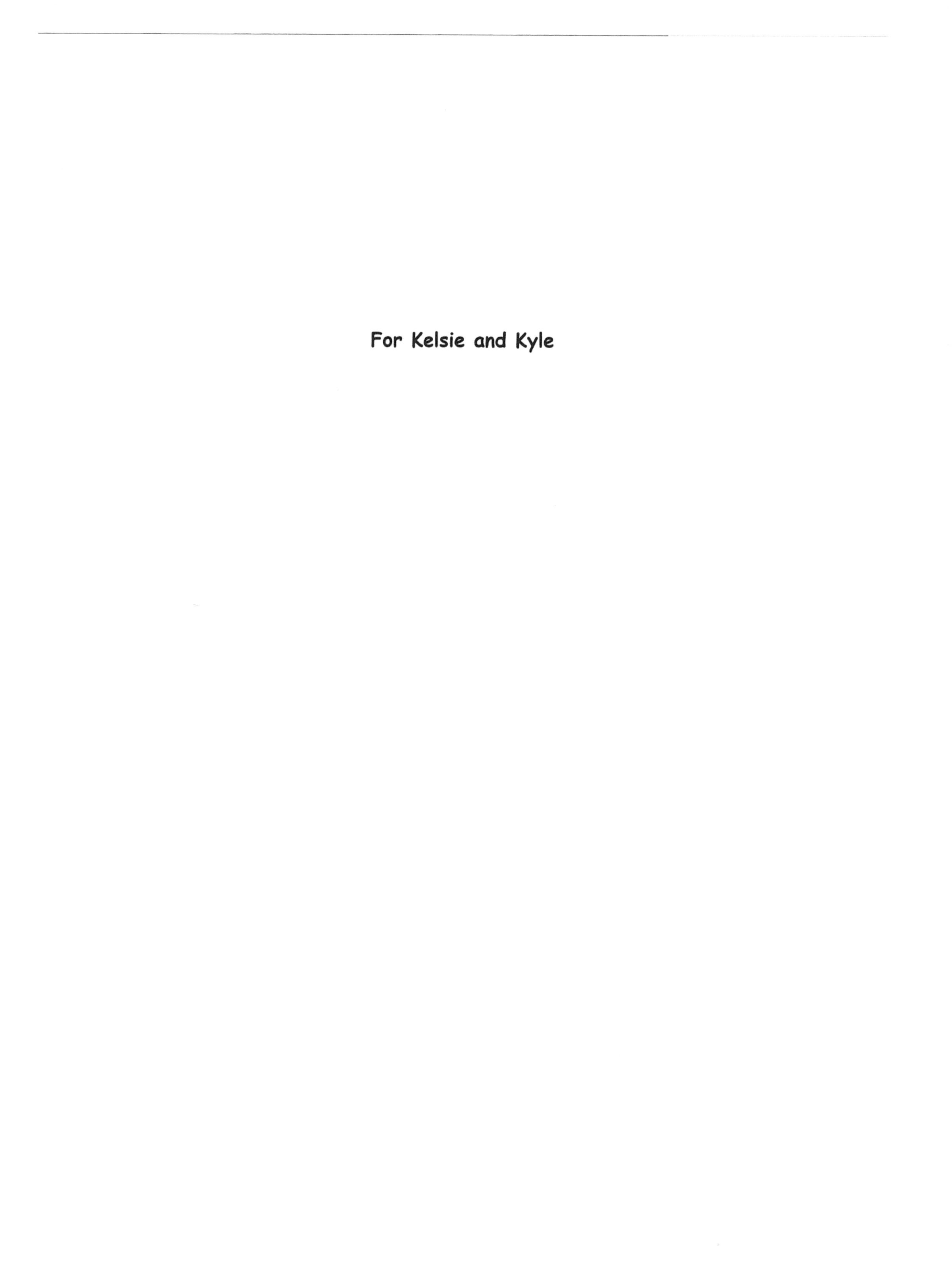

For Kelsie and Kyle

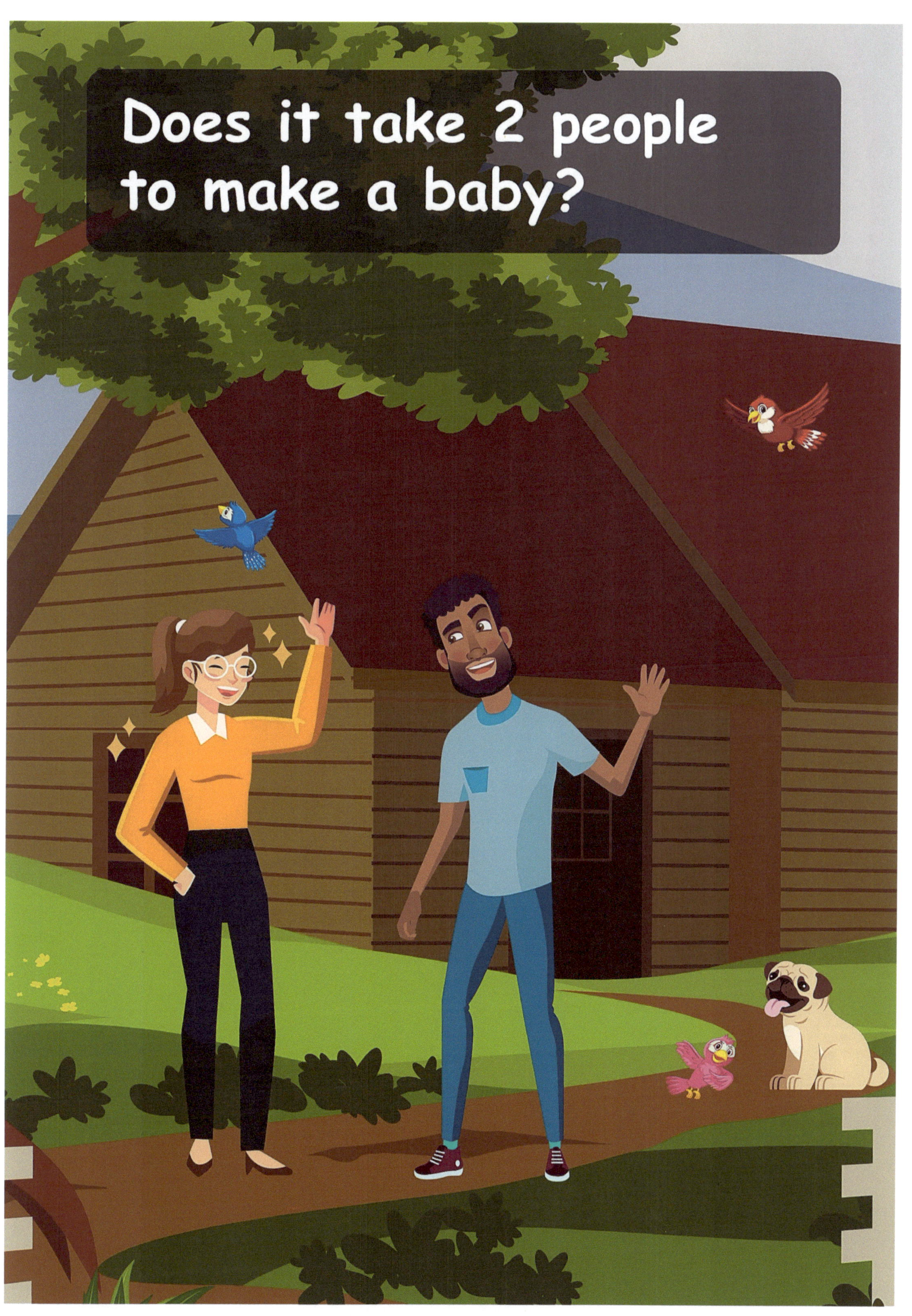
Does it take 2 people
to make a baby?

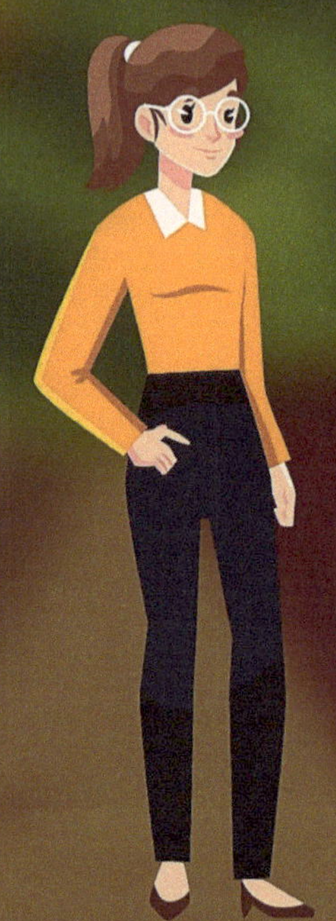
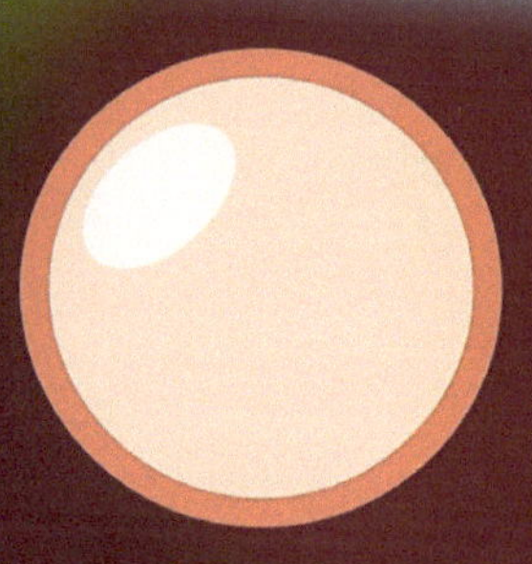

With love, the mommy gives an egg

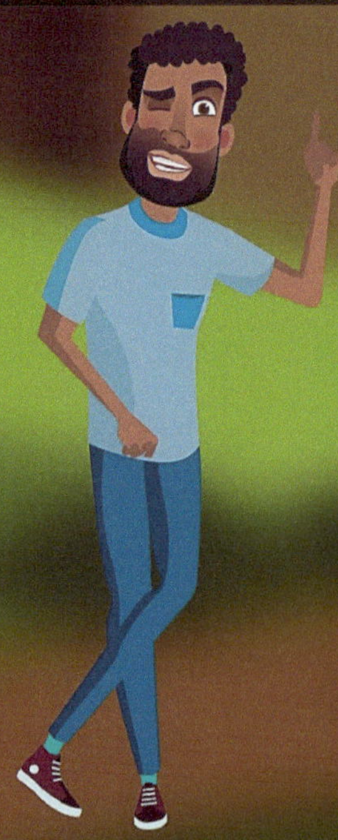
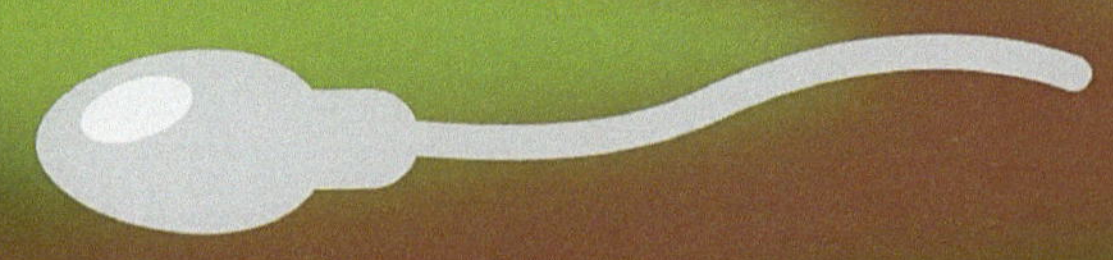

and the daddy provides sperm.

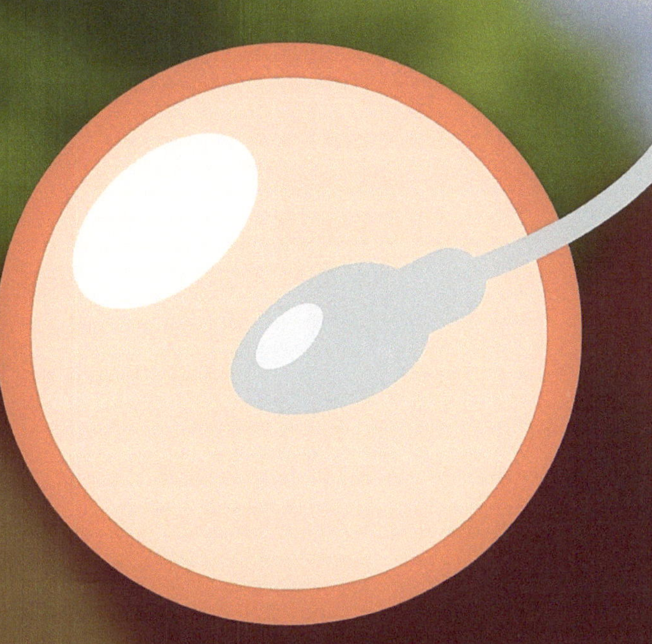
The sperm enters the egg

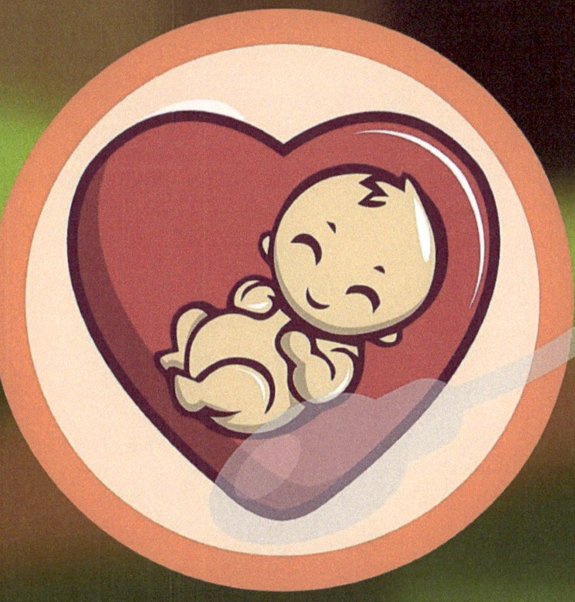
and together they form what will become a tiny baby.

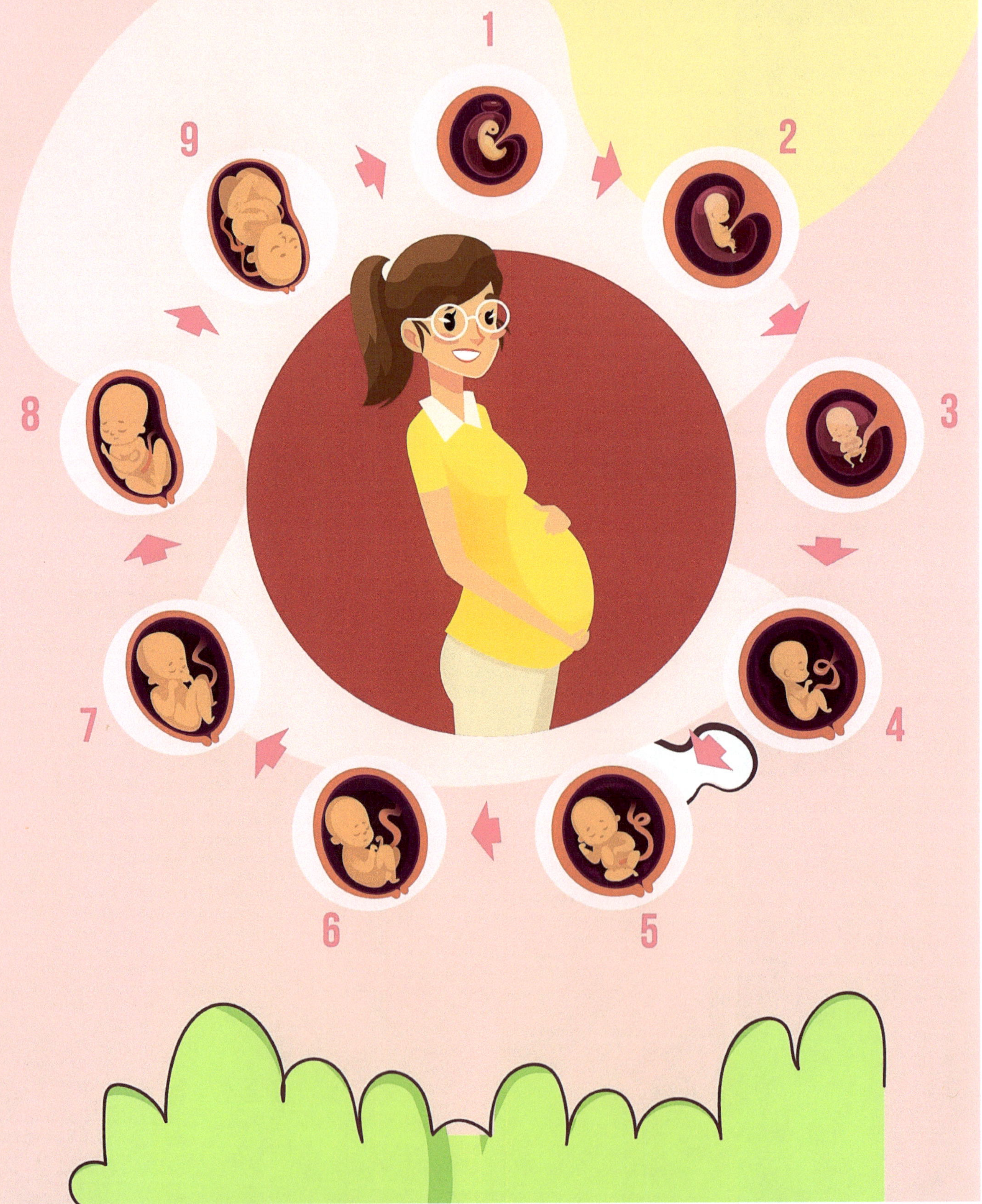
The mama's belly is a warm and safe place for the baby to grow.

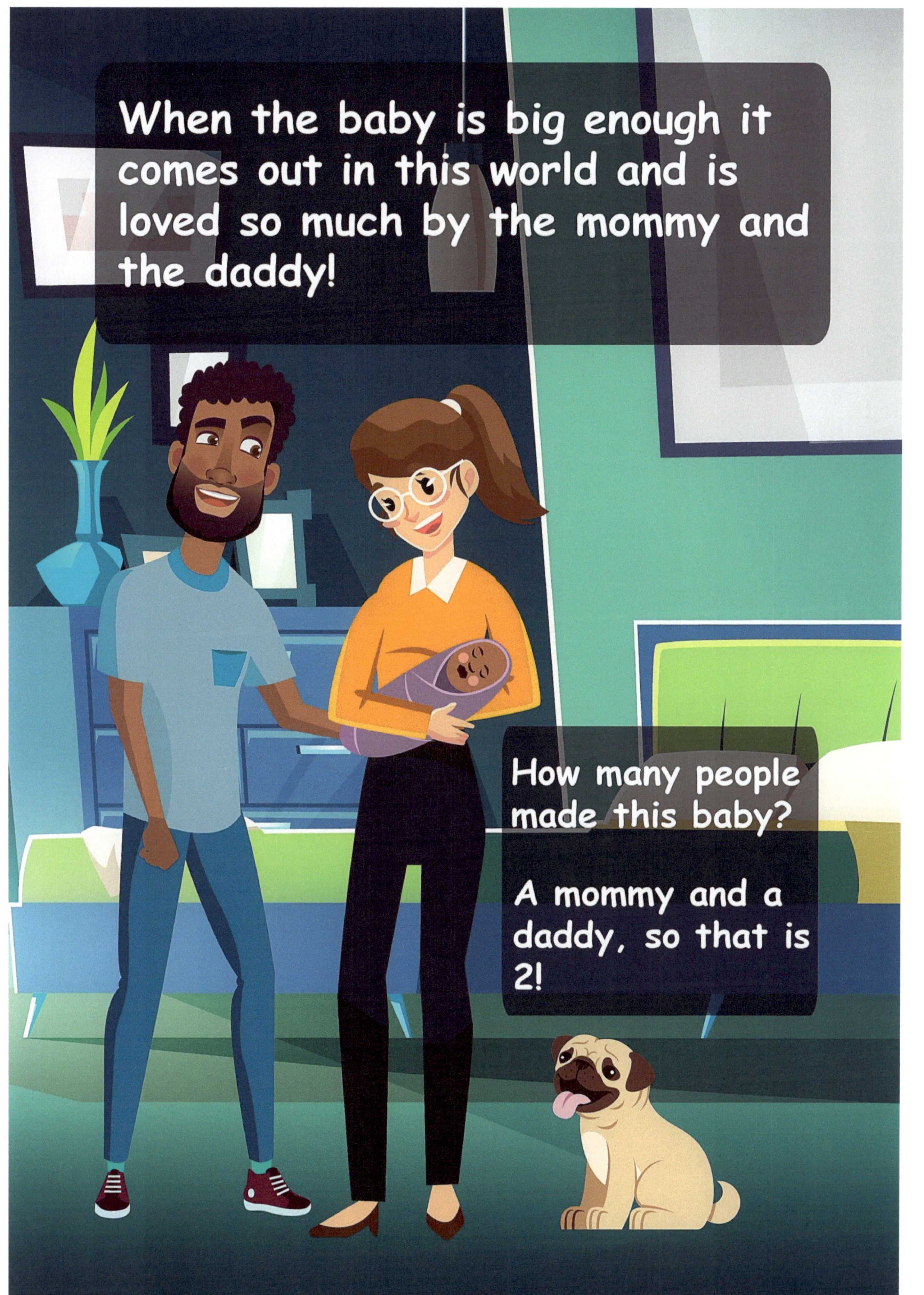
When the baby is big enough it comes out in this world and is loved so much by the mommy and the daddy!
How many people made this baby?
A mommy and a daddy, so that is 2!

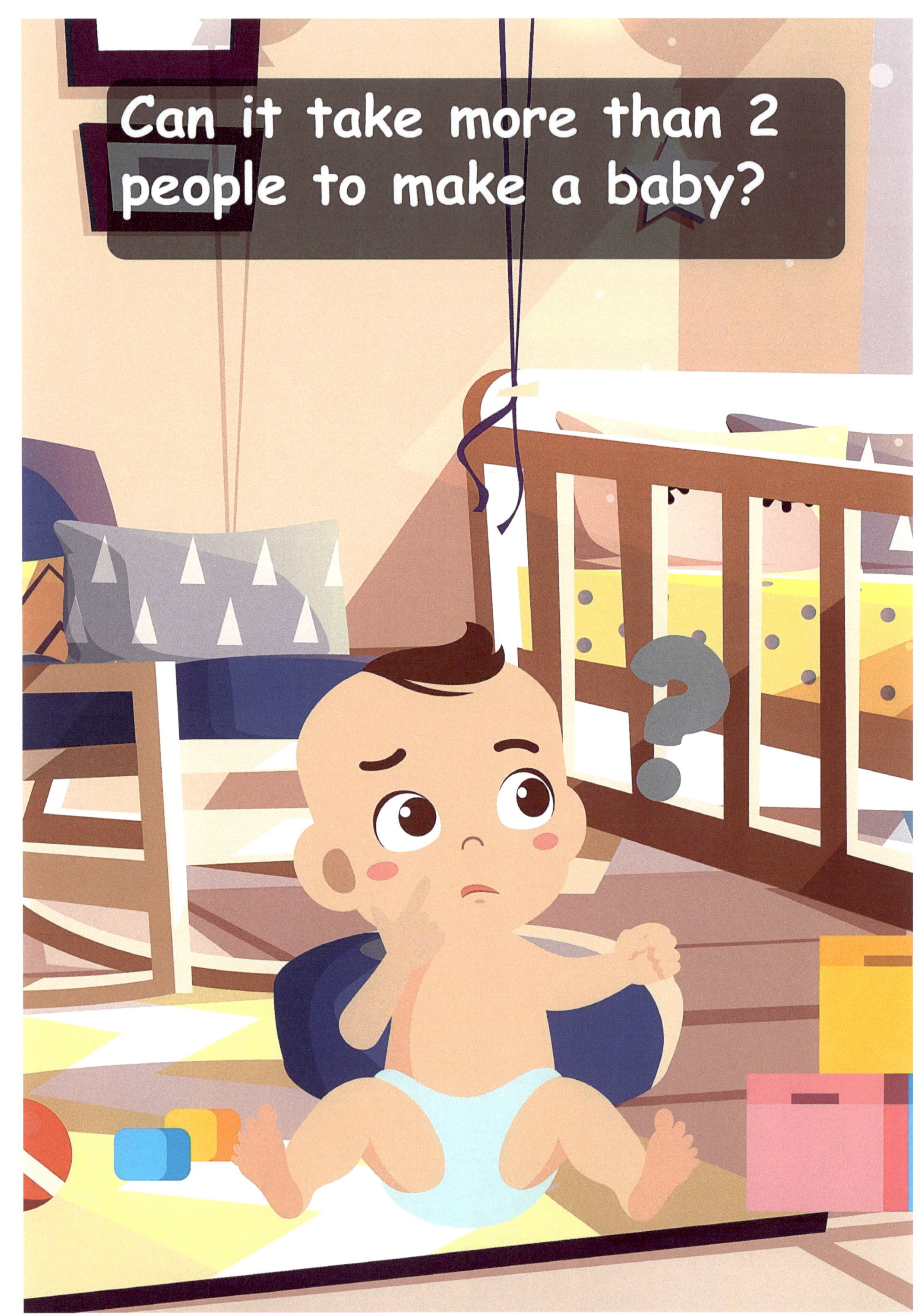
Can it take more than 2 people to make a baby?

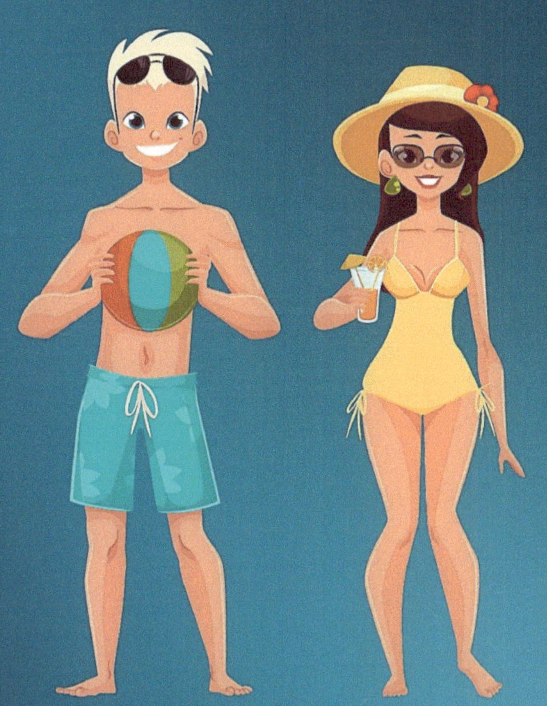

Sometimes a mommy and daddy need a little help.

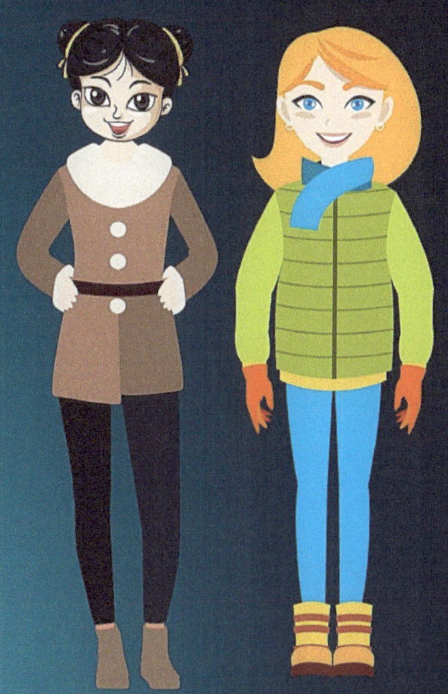

Or maybe it's two mommies that need some help.

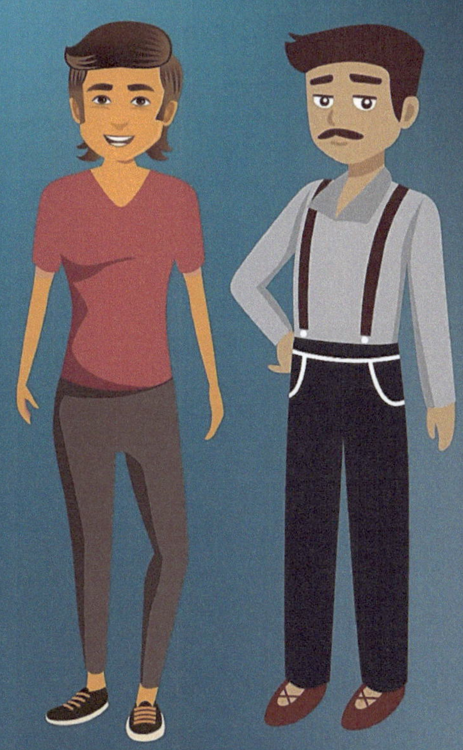

Or maybe it's two daddies.

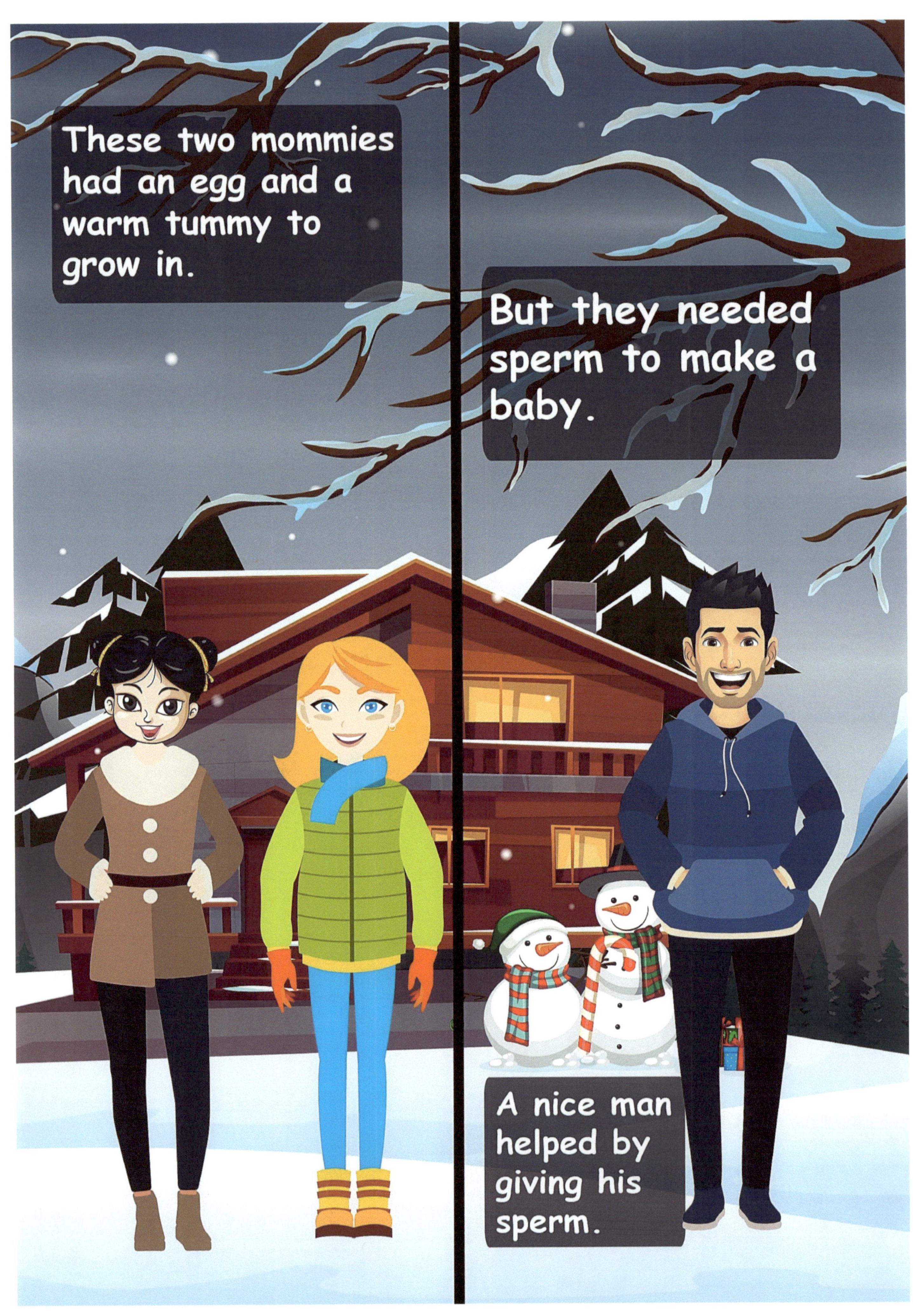

These two mommies had an egg and a warm tummy to grow in.
But they needed sperm to make a baby.
A nice man helped by giving his sperm.

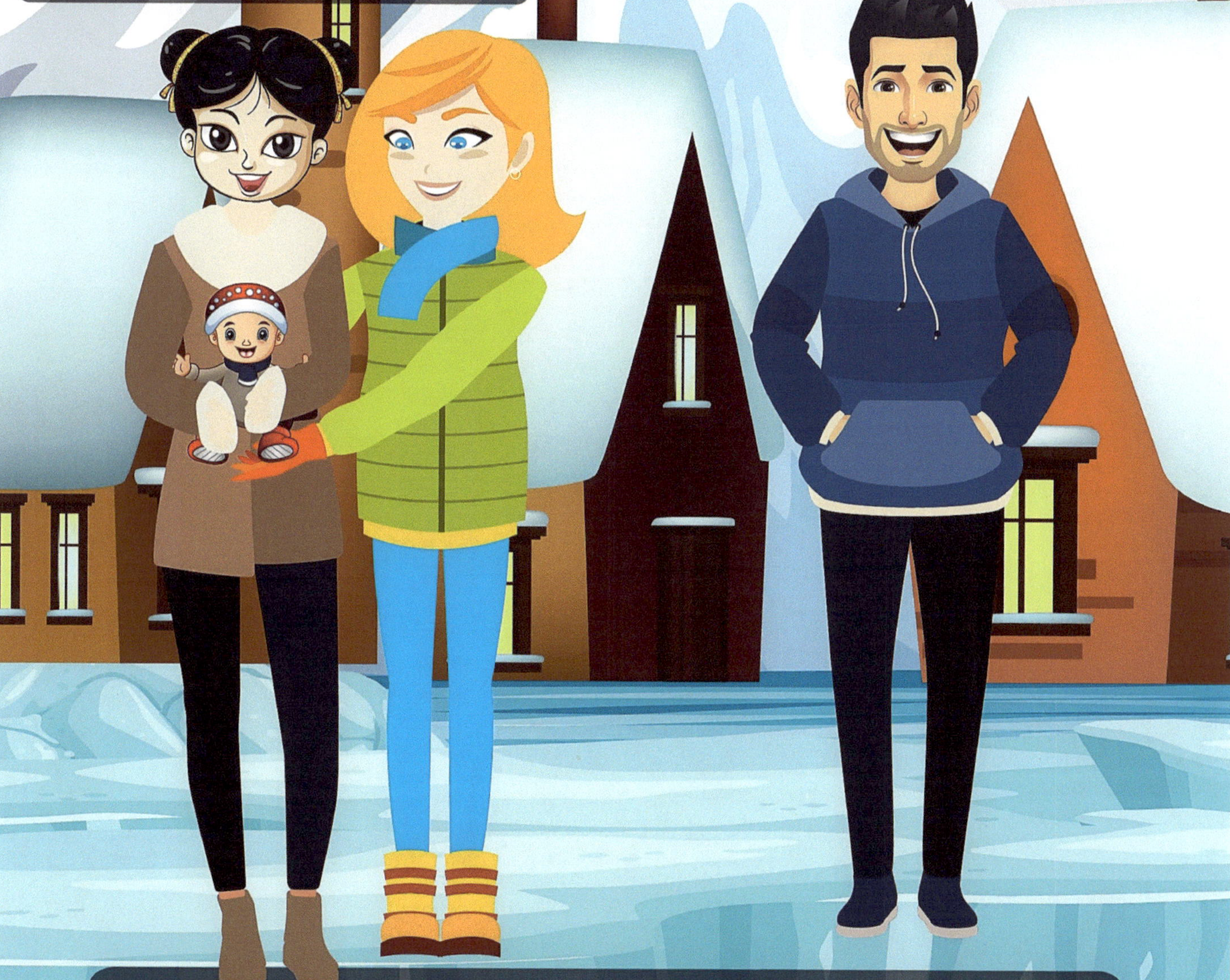

How many people did it take to make this baby?
The 2 mommies love their baby so much.
It took 2 mommies and 1 nice man. That's 3!

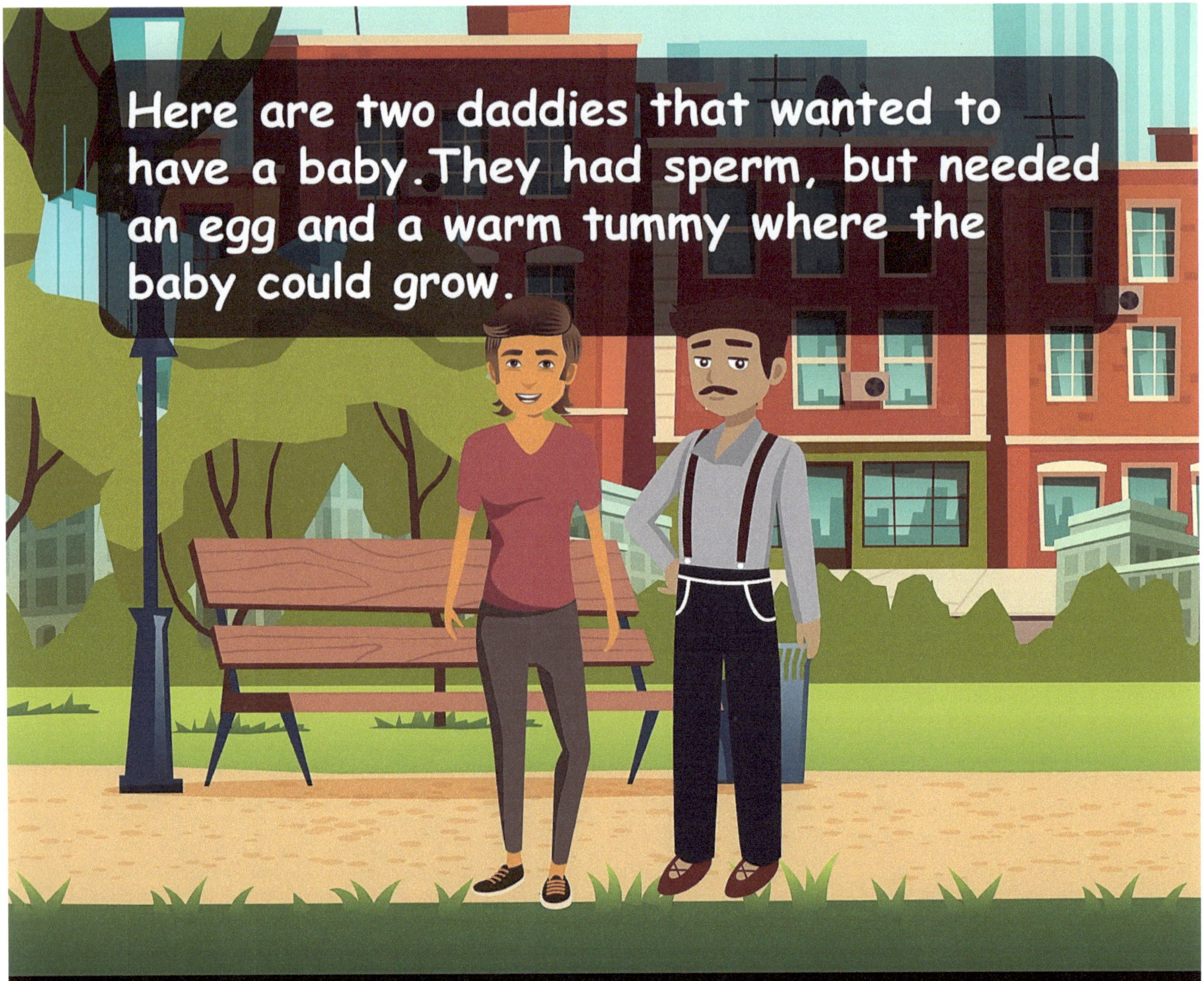

Here are two daddies that wanted to have a baby. They had sperm, but needed an egg and a warm tummy where the baby could grow.

A kind women had both the egg and warm tummy.

The sperm and egg formed a tiny baby that grew in the lady's safe and warm tummy.

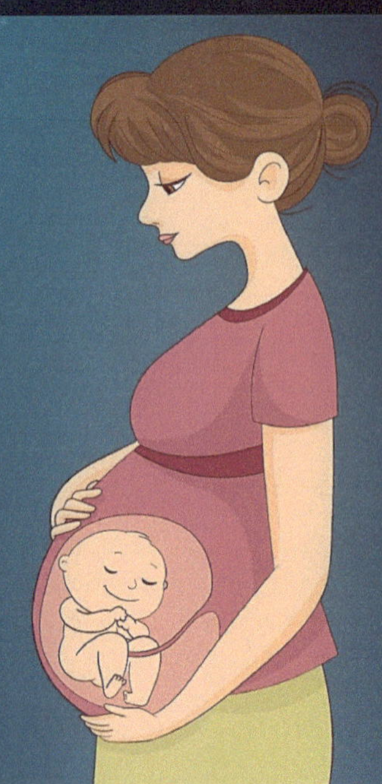

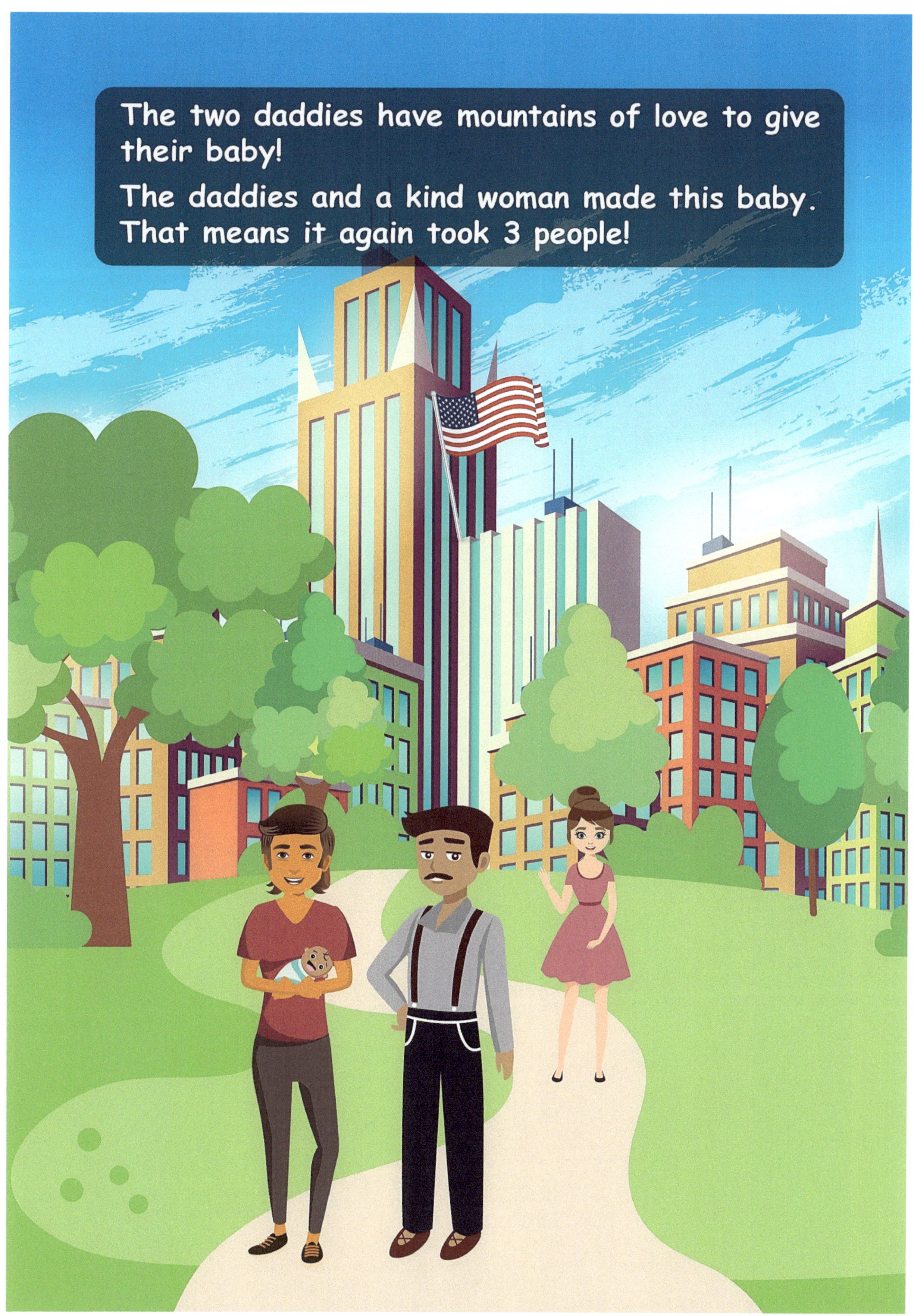

The two daddies have mountains of love to give their baby!
The daddies and a kind woman made this baby. That means it again took 3 people!

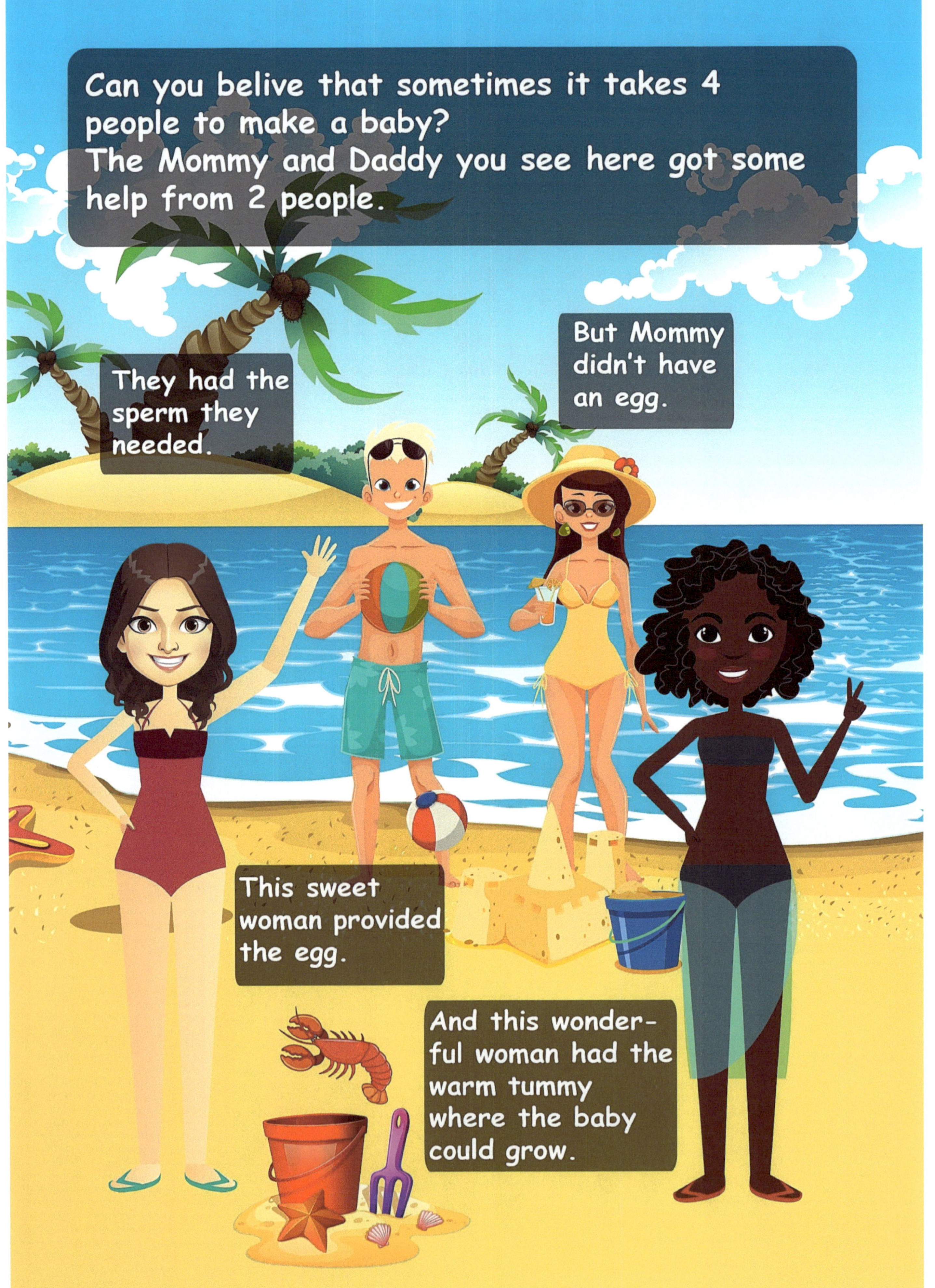

Can you belive that sometimes it takes 4 people to make a baby?
The Mommy and Daddy you see here got some help from 2 people.
They had the sperm they needed.
But Mommy didn't have an egg.
This sweet woman provided the egg.
And this wonderful woman had the warm tummy where the baby could grow.

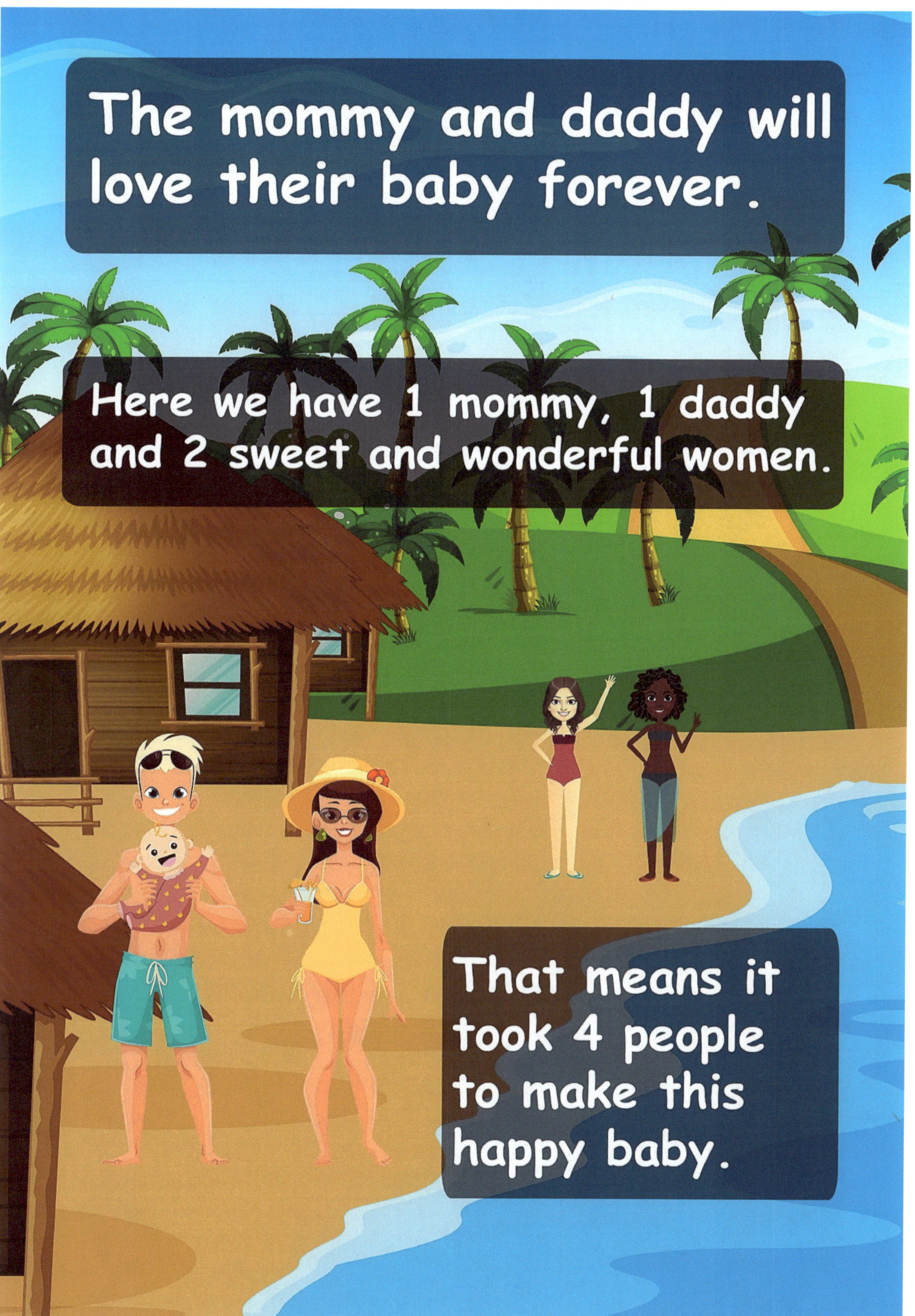

The mommy and daddy will love their baby forever.
Here we have 1 mommy, 1 daddy and 2 sweet and wonderful women.
That means it took 4 people to make this happy baby.

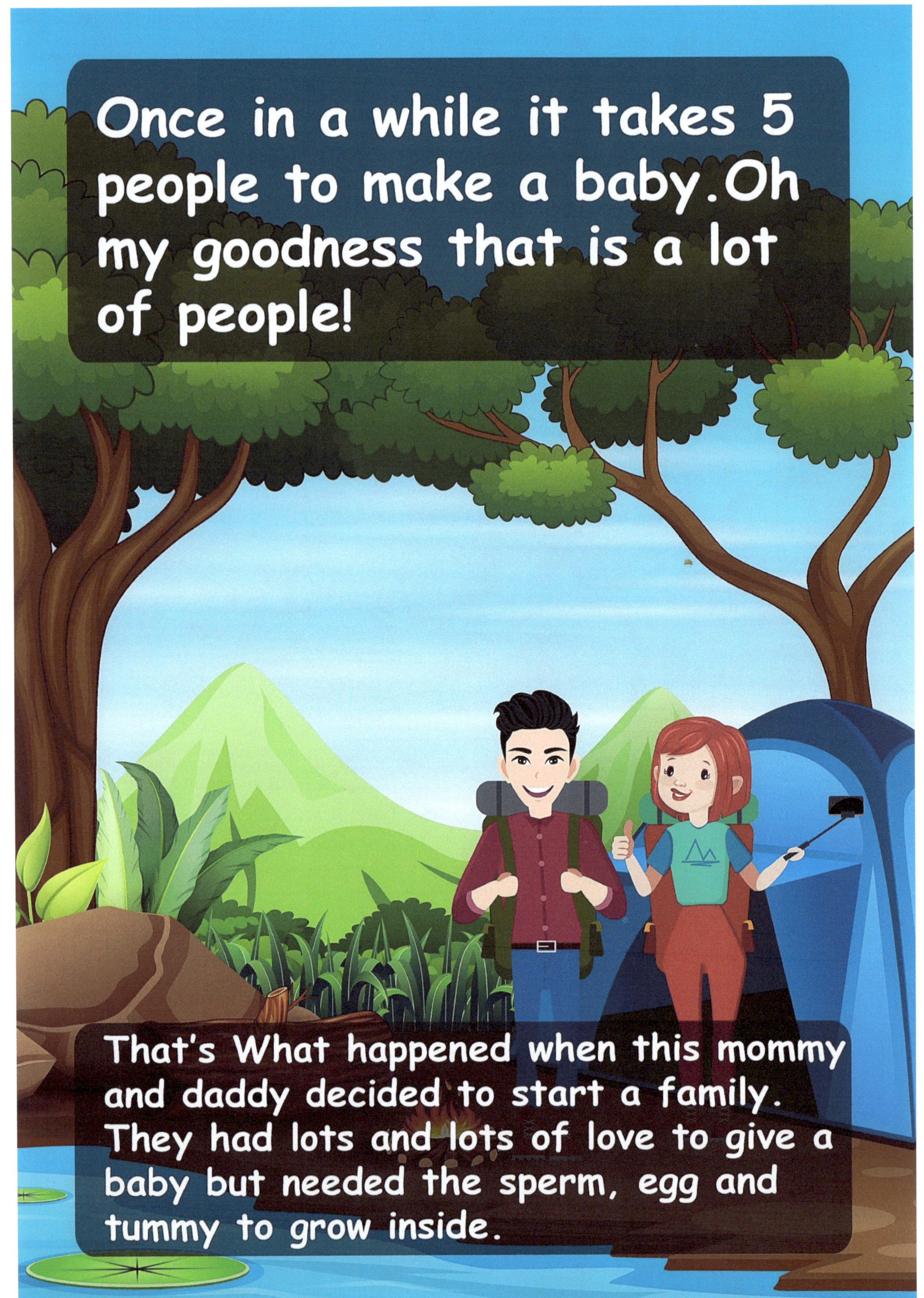
Once in a while it takes 5 people to make a baby.Oh my goodness that is a lot of people!

That's What happened when this mommy and daddy decided to start a family. They had lots and lots of love to give a baby but needed the sperm, egg and tummy to grow inside.

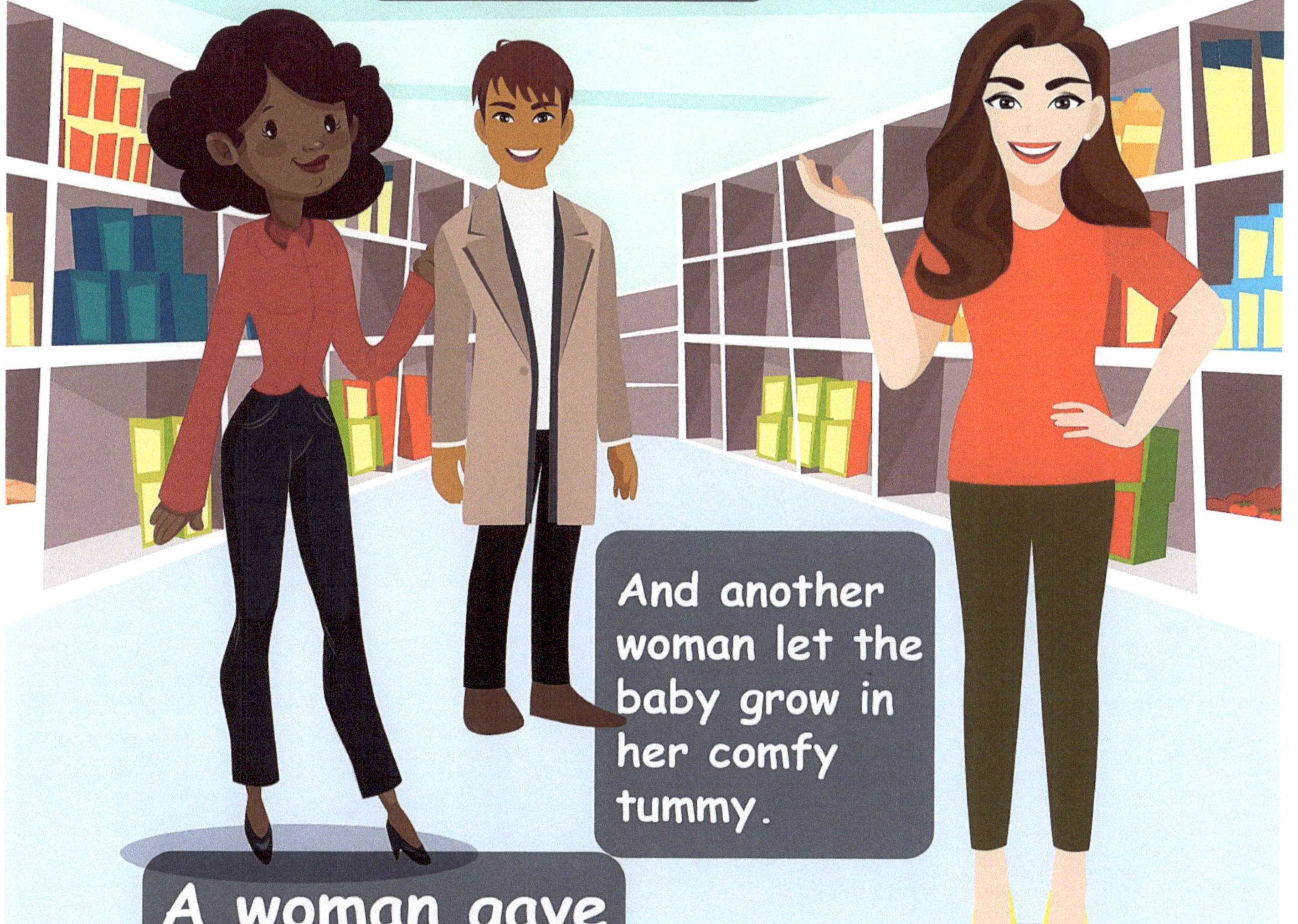

They were helped by 3 generous people.
A man gave his sperm.
And another woman let the baby grow in her comfy tummy.
A woman gave an egg.

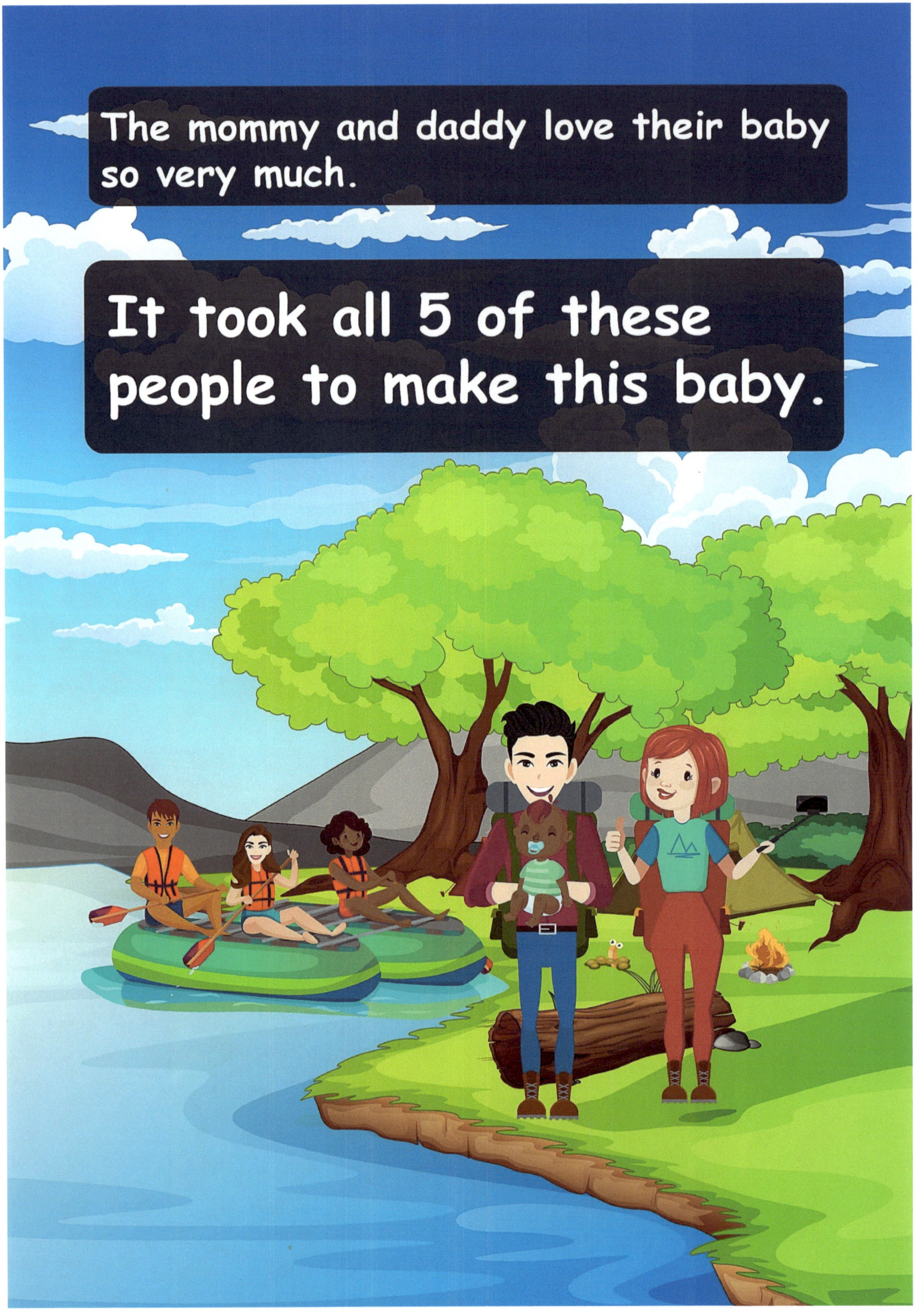

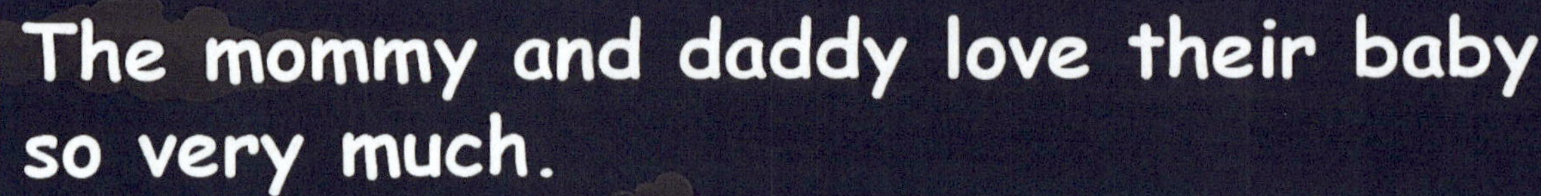

The mommy and daddy love their baby so very much.
It took all 5 of these people to make this baby.

All babies are very special and loved so much. It doesn't matter how many people it takes to make them.

You are loved to the moon and back!

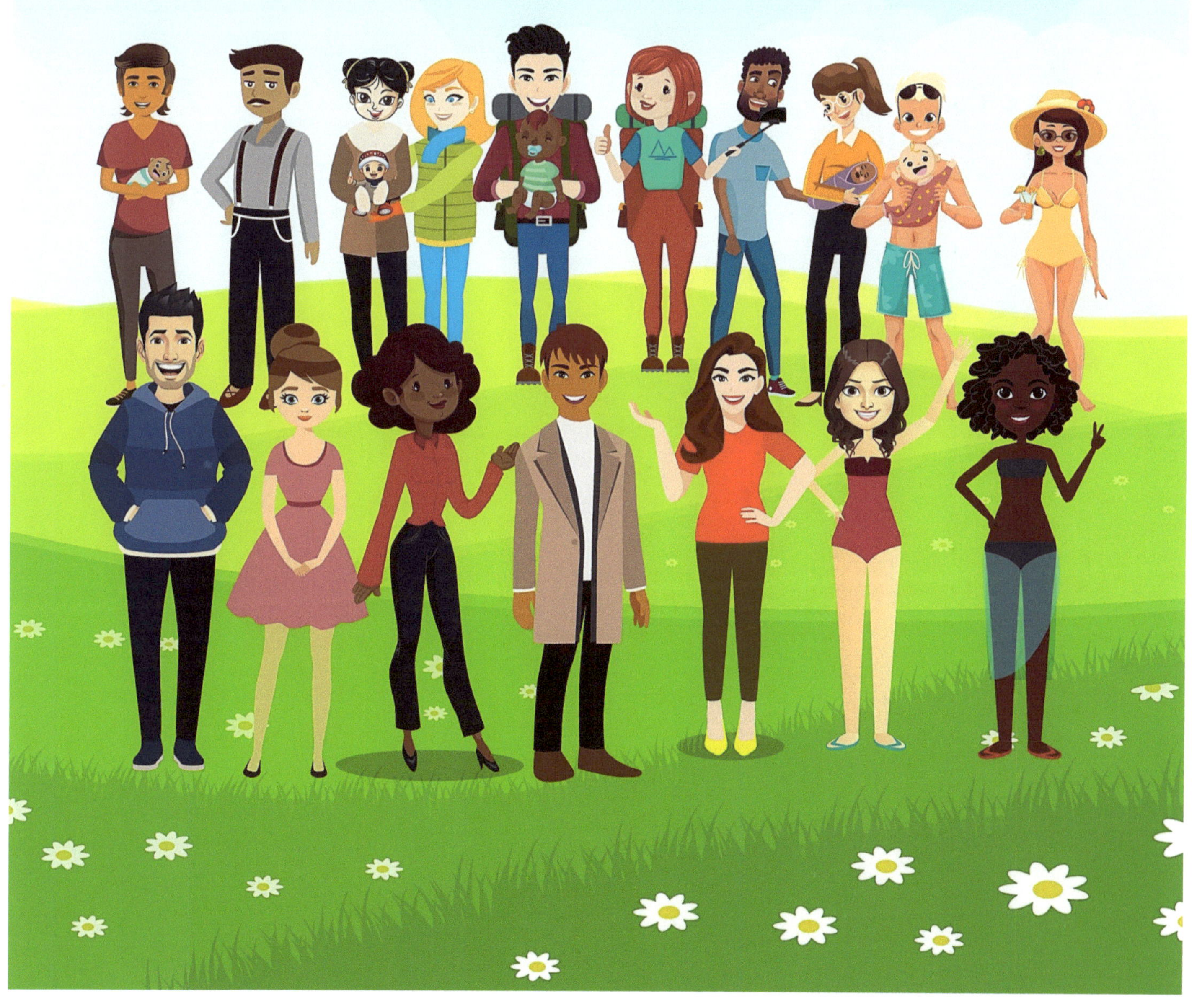

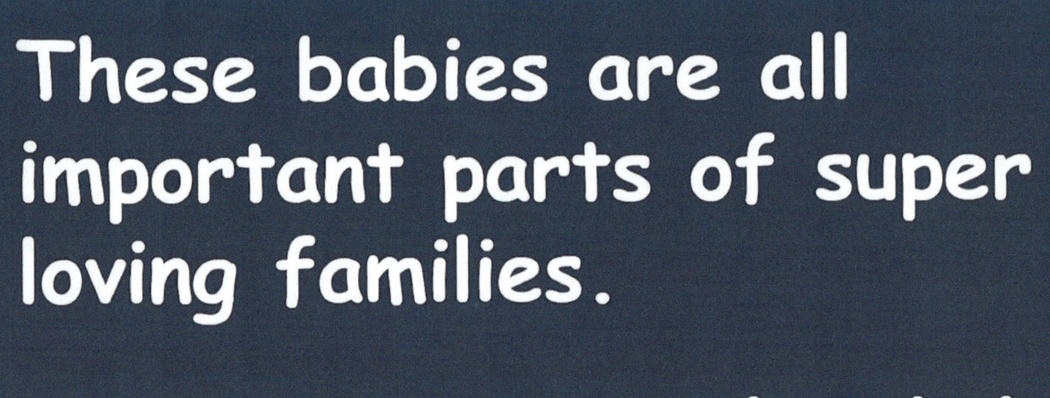

These babies are all important parts of super loving families.

How many people did it take to make you?

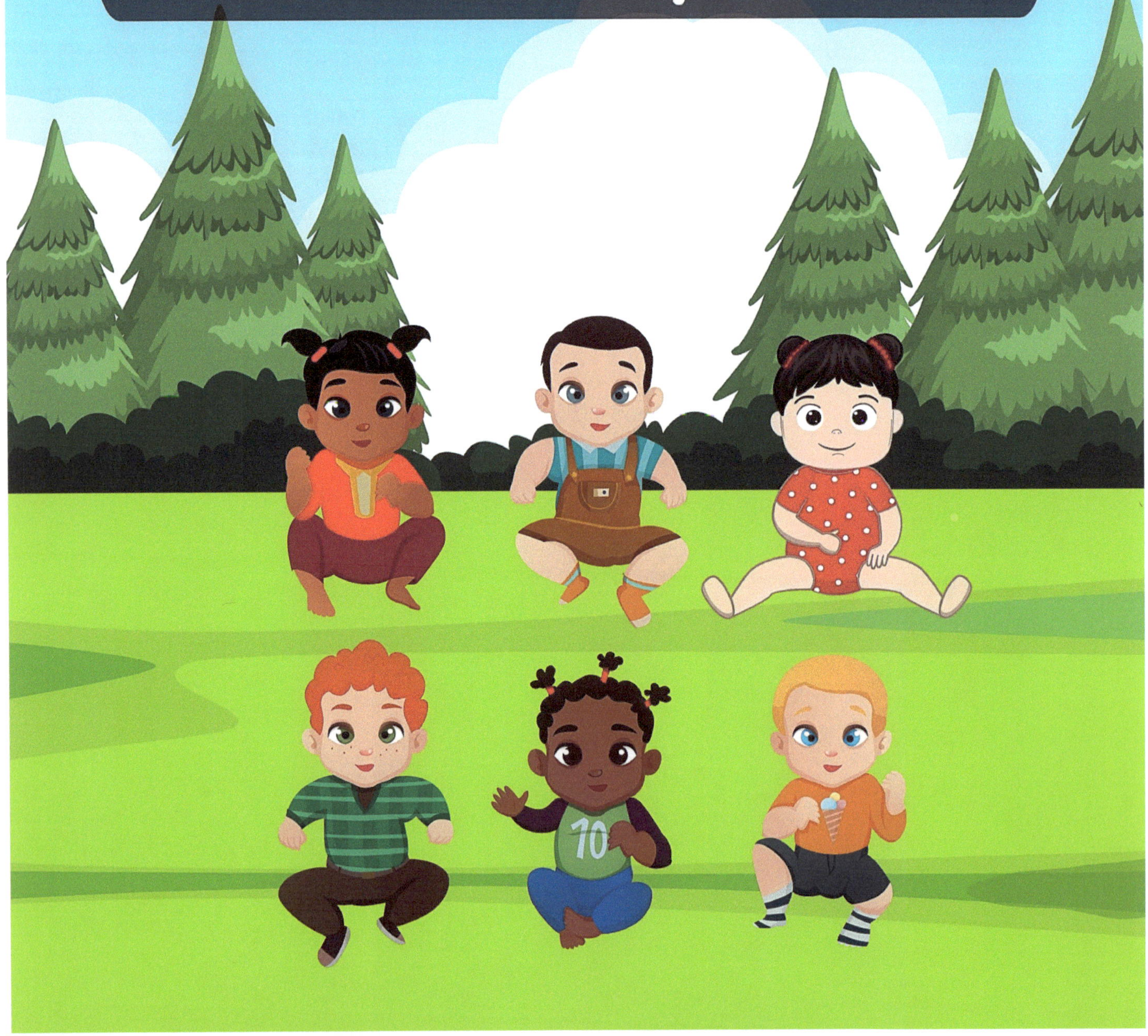